A MOTHER'S PRAYERS
WEEK BY WEEK DEVOTIONAL FOR YOUR LITTLE ONE

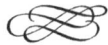

JOANNE SOJINU

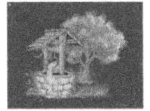

JOIN JOANNE'S READER'S LIST

Join Joanne's Reader's list for her blogs, updates on new books and free giveaways.

Please see details of how to join at the back of the book.

ISBN 978-1-9161228-1-9

Copyright © 2018 by Joanne Sojinu

First Printing—2018

The moral right of the author has been asserted

All rights reserved. No portion of this book may be reproduced, stored in a retrieval system, or transmitted in any form or by any means—electronic, mechanical, photocopy, recording, scanning or other—except for brief quotations in reviews or articles, without the prior permission of the publisher

Unless otherwise noted, all Scriptures are taken from the New King James Version® (NKJV). Copyright © 1982 by Thomas Nelson. Used by permission. All rights reserved.

Printed in the United Kingdom

Visit Authors website: Joanneswellofpearls.com

Joanne's Well Of Pearls Ltd

71-75 Shelton Street, Covent Garden, WC2H 9JQ

PART I

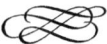

A Mother's Prayers

INTRODUCTION

A Mother's Prayers

PURPOSE

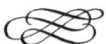

The purpose of writing this devotional is to honour expectant mothers with a resource they can use to reach out to a loving heavenly Father in prayers for the child/children they carry with a confident assurance that He hears their prayers.

Not only does the Father hear us when we pray, but He is also willing to answer our prayers.

In Luke 11:1–13, when the disciples asked Jesus to teach them how to pray, He gave them a model in the Lord's Prayer. We can build on this model; for example, using verse two, we acknowledge God as our Father in heaven and pray for His Kingdom to come and for His will to be done in the life of our unborn child or children, on earth just as He has envisioned it in heaven.

Our words can move mountains "For assuredly, I say to you, whoever says to this mountain, 'Be removed and be cast into the sea,' and does not doubt in his heart, but believes that those things he says will be done, he will have whatever he says" (Mark 11:23 NKJV).

Jesus is encouraging us through this scripture that we

have a level of authority through our spoken words that we can use, in partnership with Him, to build His kingdom and purposes on earth as it is in heaven.

The Bible gives us an example of a devoted mother who committed her son to the Lord.

Her name was Hannah, and her story can be found in 1 Samuel 1. Hannah, who had been barren, had prayed unceasingly for a child, promising to give her child to God if she could be blessed with motherhood.

After much prayer, Hannah gave birth to a healthy son, Samuel. As promised, she did commit her son's life to serving God all his days.

In turn, Samuel did go on to create a better generation than the one into which he was born. With God's guidance, Samuel commissioned strong kings to lead His people. God also gave these kings mighty men of valour, enabling them to win great battles.

Because Hannah had prayed so diligently and faithfully for Samuel, dedicating him from birth to the service of God, her story invites us to dedicate our own children to God and pray that His will and unique purpose be done in their lives.

GOD'S WORD IS POWERFUL

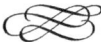

The Scripture clearly states that we have the power in our mouths to speak words of life.

We need to lay hold of that promise and speak life-giving words into our circumstance and, in this case, into the lives of our unborn children, appropriating the blessings Christ died to give us.

We must be active and not passive about this matter.

We are also encouraged to be bold and filled with the expectation that He can do the impossible, for what's impossible with man is possible with God.

God can be as awesome to us as we believe Him to be. "Therefore do not cast away your confidence, which has great reward" (Hebrews 10:35).

I would like to clarify that using this devotional should not be perceived as a legalistic route to obtain the blessings of the Lord, but because you are already blessed and highly favoured as a beloved child of God.

You are not speaking the Word of God to be blessed, but because you are already blessed and merely walking in the blessings and covering your children with them.

And even if you are not a Christian but choose to believe and read this devotional, I believe that God will honour the words you pray over your child. Every child is a gift from God, including you and your baby.

WHAT YOU WILL GET

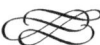

In this devotional, I explore the power of a mother's prayers. I give you the words you can use to devote your children's lives to God and to pray for divine intervention and protection for those you love most in this world.

Week by week we will walk together through the beautiful journey of pregnancy, preparing your beloved baby for a lifetime of positive choices, unshakable faith-based self-esteem, healthy coping mechanisms, and a wise and discerning mind.

Thank you for letting me be a part of this journey, and may our collective prayers begin to heal the generations to follow.

HOW TO USE THIS DEVOTIONAL

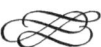

This devotional will follow the 38 weeks it takes to bring a pregnancy to term using the fertilisation age of the developing baby.

It is not usual for a woman to know exactly when she conceives within the first week of pregnancy.

Pregnancy is generally established at the date of the beginning of the last period, but technically, pregnancy doesn't occur until two weeks later, as fertilisation takes place during ovulation.

The actual timing of ovulation varies with each woman. If you have a 28-day cycle, ovulation normally occurs 14 days before your next period; therefore, this technical calculation means you're pregnant two weeks before you've actually conceived.

Averagely, a pregnancy lasts 40 weeks or 280 days from the date of your last period; to calculate your due date you count 280 days from the first day of your period and add 7 days or count 3 months back from the date of your last period and add 7 days.

This will give you an approximate due date; it is also called the gestational age or menstrual age.

The purpose of this computation is for doctors to establish the due date of the baby, so they can carry out tests at appropriate stages of the pregnancy, and women are more aware of the date of their last period than their conception date. However, keep in mind the gestational age is two weeks longer than the ovulation or fertilisation age.

The doctor will use the gestational age throughout your pregnancy, but for the purposes of using this devotional to pray at accurate growth stages of the baby, you would need to use the ovulation date.

If the gestational age of the baby is four weeks, the ovulation age would be two weeks.

As you may not know you are pregnant until you miss your next period and take a test to confirm, I would suggest that you read the prayers for week's one to eight as though you are expecting and let the prayers rest with God until conception, as no prayer is lost with God.

God spoke blessings over Abraham and his seed even before Isaac was conceived (Genesis 17:1–8). If you are not monitoring pregnancy and feel there is a chance you won't be aware you are pregnant until you are about three months pregnant, then read those weeks in advance.

OVULATION AND CONCEPTION

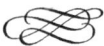

The process of ovulation takes place when one of your ovaries releases an egg, which is caught in the opening of your fallopian tube.

Pregnancy occurs when the egg is fertilised by your partner's sperm. The exact date of conception is not easy to determine, as sperm can last up to five days in the body, waiting for the release of the egg.

If no sperm is waiting, the egg continues to travel slowly along the fallopian tube.

If intercourse occurs within 24 hours of the egg being released, the egg then becomes fertilised in the fallopian tube. The moment this happens, you have conceived.

The egg, containing both yours and your partner's DNA, now becomes a single cell called the zygote. It continues to travel along the fallopian tube to the uterus, dividing as it goes but not yet growing.

With no disturbance, the zygote arrives in the uterus and implants itself within the uterine lining, making itself comfortable in a chosen spot where it will begin to grow.

At this point it becomes the embryo. This process takes seven to ten days from ovulation.

The gender and genetic makeup of the developing embryo has already been determined during fertilisation. Isn't that incredible?

As you read this devotional, visualise your unborn child inside your womb, already beloved.

CHAPTER 1

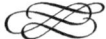

First Trimester

A Mother's Prayers

PART II

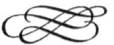

A Mother's Prayers

WEEK 0 - AGE OF YOUR LITTLE ONE

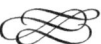

Week 1 - The First Day of Your Last Period
This is the gestation age of the child, but you have not conceived at this stage.

Your uterus begins to anticipate the coming of the baby, and the lining will thicken in order to host the baby. For calculation purposes, you are officially pregnant; however, conception takes place two weeks later.

Prayer

Heavenly Father, I thank You for providing me with a healthy womb that functions according to Your excellent design.

I pray that You would cleanse me from the inside out by the power of Your Spirit and heal me where healing is needed, so that my womb will provide a healthy and nutritious environment for my child or children.

Beloved, I pray that you may prosper in all things and be in health, just as your soul prospers (3 John 2).

WEEK 0 - AGE OF YOUR LITTLE ONE

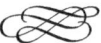

Week 2 - **From the Date of Your Last Period**
This week you're still not pregnant, but your body readies itself for ovulation. During ovulation, one of your eggs (maybe two, if twins) is released and subsequently caught in your fallopian tube, waiting to be fertilised by the sperm of your partner.

Prayer
Heavenly Father, I thank You for providing me with healthy fallopian tubes.

I pray that as fertilisation occurs in my body that You will bless and breathe life on the process so that there are healthy cell structures in my little one and that all DNA cells of myself and my partner will align according to Your excellent design with no deficiency.

Beautiful one, I praise You and bless Your holy name. Thank You for making all things new with both mine and my partner's bloodline.

Thank You that all old things have passed away, and all things have become new.

Therefore, if anyone is in Christ, he is a new creation; old things have passed away; behold, all things have become new (2 Corinthians 5:17).

WEEK 1 - AGE OF YOUR LITTLE ONE

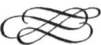

Week 1 - The Week of Conception
Week 3 - From the Date of Your Last Period

During this week, the fertilised egg travels along the fallopian tube toward the uterus, dividing as it goes but not actually growing yet.

Prayer

Awesome God, as my little one begins journeying toward the safety of my womb, may Your Spirit hover over my baby and breathe life and all Your goodness into this little one You've created. Lord, go ahead and make a way where there is no way (Isaiah 43:19).

Make every rough place smooth and do miracles where a miracle is needed. And when my little one reaches the safety of my uterus,

Lord, let my womb provide an environment of love, peace, safety, comfort, joy and healthy nourishment for Your gift of life growing inside me.

Let Your light shine in the life of this little one, whom You already knew long before, now being formed on the inside of me (2 Corinthians 4:6).

May darkness never have the power to quench the knowledge of Your light in this life growing inside my womb (John 1:5). May Your loving hands perfect this good work You've started in me and bring it to completion.

Being confident of this very thing, that He who has begun a good work in you will complete it until the day of Jesus Christ (Philippians 1:6).

WEEK 2 - AGE OF YOUR LITTLE ONE

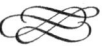

Week 2 - From the Date of Conception
Week 4 - From the Date of Your Last Period

At week two (post-fertilisation), the fertilised egg has reached the uterus and burrows into the uterine lining.

At this point, the fertilised egg becomes the embryo. Your little one is an embryo until week eight of conception. The embryo, at this stage, is a ball of cells with three main sections. In time, they will form different parts of the baby's organs.

1. The outer layer will become the neural tube and the brain, spinal cord, nerve, nose, and teeth will develop from this section.
2. The middle layer will develop into the heart, muscles, bones, and circulatory system.
3. The inner layer develops into the lungs, liver, pancreas, tongue, and gastrointestinal tract. The embryo is also rapidly dividing. In the likelihood of

identical twins, division normally occurs between days 1–13 of fertilisation.

Prayer
Gracious Lord, thank You for implanting this bundle of joy into my care.

May my body continuously provide fresh and healthy nourishment for the little one growing inside me. Hide us both under the shadow of Your mighty wings so that we will be shielded from harmful pestilence prevalent in our fallen world today (Psalm 91:6).

May the finished work of Christ on the cross begin to work newness of life into my little one's development.

May Your loving hands perfect the work You began in me. Particularly, if You have blessed me with twins, may they grow according to Your perfect design (Philippians 1:6, Psalm 138:8). I thank You, Gracious One, that You are forming my little one into Your image and likeness.

Then God said, "Let Us make man in Our image, according to Our likeness; let them have dominion over the fish of the sea, over the birds of the air, and over the cattle, over all the earth and over every creeping thing that creeps on the earth" (Genesis 1:26).

WEEK 3 - AGE OF YOUR LITTLE ONE

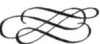

Week 3 - From the Date of Conception
Week 5 From the Date of Your Last Period
At week three, the backbone and spinal cord, the nervous system, and the brain begin formation.

Additionally, the layers of cells which develop into skin, hair, nails, nervous system, blood vessels, bones, digestive tract, and respiratory system begin to be formed.

The embryo looks like a tadpole, and cells that form various vital parts, including the spinal cord, are at work.

The heart of the embryo is formed at day 20 and starts beating at day 21 or 22 after conception.

Prayer

Heavenly Father, You are the Master Designer, and You make all things perfect and beautiful. Let Your beautiful Spirit hover over my little one as vital organs begin to form; breathe life into my baby so that every cell is perfected for development.

Thank You, Father, for giving my child a healthy brain

that is sharp and connects and coordinates well in the perfect order in which You created it to function.

I pray that my little one will have an excellent spirit and will be filled with your power, love, and a sound mind. I pray that my little one will also connect to the perfect plan You have for his/her life.

For I know the thoughts that I think toward you, says the Lord, thoughts of peace and not of evil, to give you a future and a hope (Jeremiah 29:11).

WEEK 4 - AGE OF YOUR LITTLE ONE

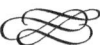

Week 4 - From the Date of Conception
Week 6 - From the Date of Your Last Period

Your little one's heart develops further and beats in a steady rhythm of 150 beats per minute. In addition to that, the arm and limb buds begin formation.

The brain is also continuing to develop as well as the beginning of the facial structure and where the eyes, nose, ears and mouth will form. Your little one's digestive tract continues to develop as well as the pancreas and spleen.

With the development of your little one's central nervous system, taking folic acid up until the 12th week facilitates the healthy development of the spinal cord. The kidney and the lungs are also developing at this stage.

Prayer

Awesome God of glory, thank You for Your magnificent work of art in the tiny body of my little one.

I pray that You will give my little one a strong and

resilient heart that will always be strong and pump life into his/her body.

Give my little one a heart that is always open to receive Your glorious grace and mercy and may his/her heart always beat with love for You and others.

May my little one's organs be fortified with health and strength to function perfectly and effectively according to Your divine order. I pray that my little one will have a healthy pancreas that will always produce insulin from now until old age.

Thank You, Father, for giving my little one a healthy spleen to fight off infections from the womb and even well into old age. May the formation of my little one be perfect.

Those who are planted in the house of the Lord
    Shall flourish in the courts of our God.
    They shall still bear fruit in old age;
    They shall be fresh and flourishing (Psalm 92:13–14).

WEEK 5 - AGE OF YOUR LITTLE ONE

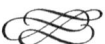

Week 5 From the Date of Conception
Week 7 From the Date of Your Last Period
During this stage, your little one's heart is further developing. Your little one's eye socket and retina begin to form, and the nasal organs appear. His or her spine continues to grow.

The hand and foot plate from which the fingers and toes grow has formed beginnings. The baby's pancreas that produces insulin continues to develop.

Nutrients and oxygen flow from you to your little one through your placenta to the umbilical cord, and also facilitate waste disposal. Your baby's kidney continues to develop. The teeth and bone cartilage are also developing.

Prayer

Dear Father of glory, at this important moment of the development of my little one, I thank You so much because I know You are present, perfecting the good work You've started in my baby's life.

Thank You for giving my little one a healthy brain that directs and coordinates all the complicated composition of the body structure. Thank You for lovely eyes that will see the world through Your eyes. Turn the eyes of my child away from worthless things.

*T*hank You for provision, sustenance, and Your Spirit that gives life more abundantly. Thank You for perfectly functioning kidneys. Thank You for a perfect pancreas that would never fail to produce insulin for my little one all the days of his/her life. Bless my little one's pancreas so that it provides healthy nutrients to him/her. Let Your Holy Spirit continue to overshadow my little one and protect him/her from the pollutions of this life.

Surely He shall deliver you from the snare of the fowler
   And from the perilous pestilence.
   He shall cover you with His feathers,
   And under His wings you shall take refuge;
   His truth shall be your shield and buckler (Psalm 91:3–4).

WEEK 6 - AGE OF YOUR LITTLE ONE

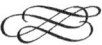

Week 6 - From the Date of Conception
Week 8 - From the Date of Your Last Period

If you're based in the UK, it is necessary for you to see your midwife or doctor for important information to assist you with having a healthy pregnancy. You would also need to book appointments for check-ups at various stages of your pregnancy.

Your little one continues to grow rapidly, and his/her sensory systems begins to develop. The beginning of the fingers and toes are developing. The baby's lungs continue to develop as well as the lymphatic system which is part of the immune system. Your little one's intestines are developing further with nerve cells.

Your little one's eyes are continuing to develop and even lids are present. Your little one's face is also forming nerve cells and taking a distinctive shape. Nerves are also forming in the legs.

Your little one's heart is beating at 150-170 beats per

minute, and your baby is making small movements. There is an increase in amniotic fluid.

Prayer

Heavenly Father and awesome Creator, thank You for the gift of life growing inside me whom You are fashioning in the dark. May my little one's hands be perfectly formed and be ever raised to give glory and honour to You.

May his/her lungs be strong and filled with breath to sing Your praises and testify of Your goodness all the days of his/her life.

May my little one have dominion over sickness and disease with the inbuilt immune system You have created so perfectly!

"For I will pour water on him who is thirsty,
   And floods on the dry ground;
   I will pour My Spirit on your descendants,
   And My blessing on your offspring" (Isaiah 44:3)

WEEK 7 - AGE OF YOUR LITTLE ONE

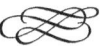

Week 7 - From the Date of Conception
Week 9 - From the Date of Your Last Period

The fetal stage of your little one is continuing its course. The arms and legs begin to grow longer as do the cartilage and bone, the taste buds, the inner ears, the lungs, the liver, the thyroid glands, the pancreas, and the hair follicles.

Your little one's digestive tract is also developing further, as well as the intestines. The baby's hands, feet, and toes are also developing.

There is limb movement that you won't feel yet. Your baby's genitals are also formed at this stage. Your little one is looking more like a baby. Isn't that wonderful!

Prayer

Heavenly Father, may the development of my baby's arms and legs be perfect to carry out Your will and walk along Your paths that are faithful and true. Breathe the breath of life into my baby's organs as they form. May they grow strong and healthy.

May my little one's digestive tract work perfectly and be free of all allergies and disorders. I thank You, Father, that You are creating healthy structures in my little one's system. (Psalm 22:9-10). Thank You also that the effective fervent prayer of the righteous man avails much (James 5:16).

Now this is the confidence that we have in Him, that if we ask anything according to His will, He hears us. And if we know that He hears us, whatever we ask, we know that we have the petitions that we have asked of Him (1 John 5:14–15).

WEEK 8 - AGE OF YOUR LITTLE ONE

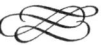

Week 8 - From the Date of Conception
Week 10 - From the Date of Your Last Period

At this stage, your little one's nose and lips begin forming as well as the tongue and larynx, fingers and toes.

Additionally, the formation of the heart is complete and functioning. The baby's eyelids are currently shut, but will open at the 28th week.

Also developing are the elbows, toes, fingers, and thumbs. The baby's teeth also begin forming under the gums. Your little one weighs around four grams and is very active, but you won't feel this movement yet. The embryonic age of your little one ends this week.

Prayer

Awesome God, thank You for the development of my baby at this stage. May my little one be perfected to commune with You and sing praises of Your great works.

May my little one's heart connect with Your purpose and destiny for his/her life. Thank You, Father, for the perfect formation of all my baby's vital parts.

**Out of the mouth of babes and nursing infants
You have ordained strength (Psalm 8:2).**

WEEK 9 - AGE OF YOUR LITTLE ONE

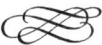

Week 9 - From the Date of Conception
Week 11 - From the Date of Your Last Period

At this stage, your little one's development is making rapid progress. The neck is gaining strength, and the baby's tiny legs are performing kicks. If the little one is a girl, her ovaries will be forming.

The external genitalia are visible, but the gender won't be known until later. Your little one's mouth, tongue, and palate are formed as well as the fingers and the toenail area. Development of the iris has begun.

The digestive tract has completed development while the brain continues to mature. Your little one's facial bones are also now complete.

Prayer

Heavenly Father, thank You for the development of this precious life that You are forming in my womb.

I thank You that You are indeed a God whom I can trust to perfect that which has been committed into Your hands.

I am connecting to Your awesome faith that You will give my little one excellent vision, healthy gums, and hands that are quick to do good. Thank You for eliminating all forms of allergies from my little one's digestive system.

Thank You for blessing my little one with a perfectly functioning brain. May my little one be well-balanced and connected to the unique treasures You have deposited in him/her and not be swayed by the deception that prevails in this world or accept anything other than Your original design for his/her life.

The Lord will perfect that which concerns me;
   Your mercy, O Lord, endures forever;
   Do not forsake the works of Your hands (Psalm 138:8).

WEEK 10 - AGE OF YOUR LITTLE ONE

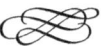

Week 10 - From the Date of Conception
Week 12 - From the Date of Your Last Period
At this stage the formation of all your little one's vital parts has been completed, and the baby begins to grow in length. The pancreas is functioning well and producing insulin.

Your little one floats around kicking, eagerly testing out his or her muscles. The baby also begins to suck his or her thumb and sometimes cries silently. Your little one can also feel pain.

Your little one's eyelids are shut for protection and will reopen around week 28. The cartilage in the skeletal structure is now forming into bone, which will take a couple of decades to fully harden. Your little one's digestive system can contract well to digest food and pass waste. Your little one now looks more like a baby. How awesome!

. . .

Prayer

Heavenly Father, I am continuously thankful for the work of artistry and excellence in this bundle of joy that You have put into my loving care. May my little one know freedom and joy with absolutely no limits within the power of Your grace (2 Corinthians 3:17).

May my womb continue to provide an environment of safety and rich nurture so that s/he may be strong and confident to grow in the world and make wise choices that lead to freedom and abundant life (John 10:10). I pray that I will produce enough nutrients to enable my little one to develop strong and healthy bones.

**Like arrows in the hand of a warrior,
So are the children of one's youth (Psalm 127:4).**

CHAPTER 2

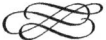

Second Trimester - Chapter 2

A Mother's Prayers

PART III

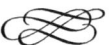

A Mother's Prayers

WEEK 11 - AGE OF YOUR LITTLE ONE

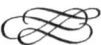

Week 11 - **From the Date of Conception**
Week 13 - From the Date of Your Last Period

At this stage, you are in your second trimester. Your little one's eyes and ears have moved to their correct position.

Additionally, you can now tell the gender of the baby through ultrasound. Bone has developed over the cartilage.

Your little one can also open and close his/her mouth and is swallowing nutritional amniotic fluid that is digested, passed, and ingested again.

The baby's intestine has moved from the umbilical cord into the abdominal cavity in preparation for the first stool.

Your little one now has his or her own fingerprints, which will further develop. The vocal cords are now developed and can make sounds that you won't hear until birth.

If you are carrying a boy, his testicles are formed as well as the penis. If you are carrying a girl, her ovaries are formed and contain around a million eggs.

. . .

Prayer

Father of glory, I give blessing, glory, and honour to Your name for the works of Your hands which my soul knows so well. Thank You for perfect hearing in my little one as s/he is being formed in Your image and likeness.

May my little one's ears hear You when You knock on the door of his/her heart, and with a willing heart, follow Your guidance through the voyage of life. I pray that my little one will have strong bones and, like Caleb, still take mountains for You in old age.

I pray that no arthritis or other bone disease will descend from my inherited genes to touch my little one. For through the love of Christ and His finished work on the cross, He has made all things new. Thank You for the redeeming power of the cross (Galatians 3:13). I pray my little one's reproductive system will be healthy and will produce healthy children under Your care when the time comes.

Behold, I stand at the door and knock. If anyone hears My voice and opens the door, I will come in to him and dine with him, and he with Me (Revelation 3:20).

WEEK 12 - AGE OF YOUR LITTLE ONE

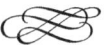

Week 12 - From the Date of Conception
Week 14 - From the Date of Your Last Period

At this stage, your little one has developed a full-body coat of soft hair for warmth. This pale fur will shed naturally, generally before birth. Eyebrows have also formed. Your little one's limbs are developing further and making coordinated movements. Your little one is also flexing facial muscles to display a variety of expressions.

The baby's mouth is fully formed and is practising the swallowing movement. Your baby's neck is becoming stronger to maintain an upright position.

***P**rayer*

Precious Lord of glory, I give You ceaseless thanks for the continuous development of my little one. May Your gracious and loving hands be upon my child and may the light of Your glory shine around my child.

May my little one be full of life, vigour, and vitality. May s/he be aligned to live according to Your original design through and through. May the light of Your glory shine in and through my little one

---

> But we all, with unveiled face, beholding as in a mirror the glory of the Lord, are being transformed into the same image from glory to glory, just as by the Spirit of the Lord (2 Corinthians 3:18).

WEEK 13 - AGE OF YOUR LITTLE ONE

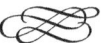

Week 13 - From the Date of Conception
Week 15 - From the Date of Your Last Period

At this stage, your little one's legs are still growing. Though you may not feel them yet, s/he is making reflexive movements with his/her arms and legs.

Your little one is able to hear sounds coming from both inside and outside the womb, and is also able to see light through his/her eyes that are not yet open.

The bones are getting stronger; Your little one is also practising breathing while still floating in the amniotic fluid.

Prayer

Gracious God, I thank You that You, the One who neither slumbers nor sleeps, are watching over the development of my little one.

Thank You for every movement of my child; I pray that my little one's ears will be open to hear Your gentle loving voice and be forever secure in Your steadfast love and may his/her feet be willing to follow You along the paths of righteousness.

Thank You for strengthening my little one's bones. Thank You for perfect, healthy skin.

"**Fear not, for I am with you;**
   Be not dismayed, for I am your God.
   I will strengthen you,
   Yes, I will help you,
   I will uphold you with My righteous right hand"
(Isaiah 41:10).

WEEK 14 - AGE OF YOUR LITTLE ONE

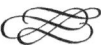

Week 14 - From the Date of Conception
Week 16 - From the Date of Your Last Period

At this stage, your little one is growing more rapidly, and his/her muscles are getting stronger. Your little one can hold his or her hands together and may even be able to suck his/her tongue.

Your little one's nerve connections are in full function, enabling reflex movements. You may start to feel this movement, which may feel like little flutters.

Prayer

Dear Lord, thank You for developing my little one into a strong and healthy baby. Thank You for Your keen eye of watch and care over my little one, as his/her intricate parts grow and function according to Your perfect design.

I pray that my little one's nervous system will be healthy and that s/he will be free to do all the things You've predestined him/her to do.

Lord, please help me to overcome the fear associated with my body changing, and instead help me to turn my eyes towards you, and the joy of this beautiful gift of life you have blessed me with.

Behold, the eye of the Lord is on those who fear Him, On those who hope in His mercy (Psalm 33:18).

WEEK 15 - AGE OF YOUR LITTLE ONE

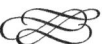

Week 15 - From the Date of Conception
Week 17 - From the Date of Your Last Period

Your baby begins to develop fat under the skin to keep the body warm after birth and may also be developing sweat glands under the thin transparent skin.

The placenta continues to grow and provide essential nutrients to your little one.

Your baby's toes and fingerprints have also formed their unique print.

Prayer

Loving Father, thank You for Your blessings that are new every morning. I pray that the placenta will grow healthy and so that my little one can receive abundant nutrition from all the foods I eat to support his/her growth.

I pray that my little one develops healthy skin to keep him/her warm after birth, in Jesus' name. I thank You, Lord, that You are surrounding my baby with favour like a shield as s/he rests under the shadow of Your mighty wings (Psalm 91:1-4).

For You, O Lord, will bless the righteous;
   With favour You will surround him as with a shield (Psalm 5:12).

WEEK 16 - AGE OF YOUR LITTLE ONE

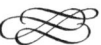

Week 16 - From the Date of Conception
Week 18 - From the Date of Your Last Period

If you're based in the UK, you are offered an ultrasound scan between weeks 18-20, to check the development of your little one.

At this stage, your little one is developing myelin, a protective substance formed around the nerve fibres of the nervous system to insulate it.

Your little one is becoming very active, kicking, somersaulting, and rolling. Your little one has also learned to yawn and hiccup.

His/her vocal cords have developed as well. S/he has also developed vernix caseosa, a skin coating which preserves the condition of the baby's skin whilst in amniotic fluid.

Prayer

Heavenly Father, thank You for the miracle of life that is steadily growing in my womb.

I thank You that You are continuously watching over my little one as You are perfecting the work You've started. Thank You for healthy vocal cords that will work perfectly according to Your original design.

Thank You for giving my little one beautiful skin, perfect lungs, and the grace You've given my little one as s/he exercises his/her lungs.

May they be healthy and strong to join us in singing praises as we behold the glorious works of Your hands (Psalm 92:4-5; 139:14). Thank You for filling my little one with joy, peace, and lots of fun. Thank You for giving me strength and good health to bring my little one safely to full term.

I can do all things through Christ who strengthens me
   (Philippians 4:13).

WEEK 17 - AGE OF YOUR LITTLE ONE

Week 17 - From the Date of Conception
Week 19 - From the Date of Your Last Period

If your little one is a girl, her female reproductive organs will have formed at this stage; if the little one is a boy, his genitals will have formed and are visible during a scan.

The translucency will have disappeared from your baby's skin as s/he will have developed pigmentation.

Your little one has developed sensors to hear distinctive sounds more clearly as well as the senses of taste, smell, and sight. Your little one can even sense your stress.

Prayer

Creator of heaven and earth, thank You for blessing my little one and for planting the seeds of procreation within his/her body.

Breathe the breath of life, grace, and favour into those seeds that would carry through from generation to generation. May my little one honour You with his/her body and may the seed of my little one know no corruption (Psalm 112:2).

I pray that Your peace rules in my heart so that I am not passing down stress to my little one. Protect my precious little one so that s/he only receives all the good things needed for development. May my womb be a place of sanctity, peace, love, joy, and nourishment for my little one

---

"Peace I leave with you, My peace I give to you; not as the world gives do I give to you. Let not your heart be troubled, neither let it be afraid" (John 14:27).

WEEK 18 - AGE OF YOUR LITTLE ONE

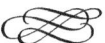

Week 18 - From the Date of Conception
Week 20 - From the Date of Your Last Period

Your little one is growing bigger in size but still has ample room to continue with rolling and somersaulting.

You will be able to feel the movements more distinctly as your baby has grown bigger and stronger.

The milk teeth have formed at this point, and the permanent ones will start to bud, all below the gums.

The nerves in your little one are still developing and making connections with the brain.

Prayer

Loving Father, thank You for the continuous development of the life that You have entrusted in my care. Thank You that You are watching over the growth of his/her nervous system.

May Your fragrance of grace and love fill the senses of my

little one so that s/he will forever be familiar with and rooted in Your love and not be sold short of it.

Thank You for a strong and healthy nervous system that will know to lean on You for strength against the harsh winds of life.

I will lift up my eyes to the hills —
    From whence comes my help?
    My help comes from the Lord,
    Who made heaven and earth.
    He will not allow your foot to be moved;
    He who keeps you will not slumber
    (Psalm 121:1–3).

WEEK 19 - AGE OF YOUR LITTLE ONE

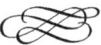

Week 19 - From the Date of Conception
Week 21 - From the Date of Your Last Period

At this stage, your little one's digestive system enables him/her to swallow small amounts of amniotic fluid, forming his/her first stool, which is stored in the bowel and passed at birth.

The process of swallowing amniotic fluid also helps with the development of the air sacs in your little one's lungs.

Also, his/her taste buds continue to develop.

There is an increase in body fat to keep your baby warm after birth. The production of white blood cells by his/her bone marrow will help fight infection.

The vernix substance has now covered the baby's body, protecting the skin in the amniotic fluid and will also be a lubricant during delivery.

. . .

Prayer

Awesome God of glory, I am again giving You thanks for the perfect development of this bundle of joy You've given me.

Thank You that Your Spirit of grace dwells on the inside of me, and therefore my life is filled with the light of Your glory; because You are in me, my little one is filled with Your light as well.

Thank You for the heart of my little one that is growing stronger day by day.

Thank You for my little one's bone marrow that is functioning according to Your perfect design and will continue to do so all the days of my baby's life. Thank You for strengthening my womb and muscles for the time of delivery.

Thank You for the vernix substance that will make the delivery easier.

Thank You, Father, that You are in total control and will be with us in the hour of labour and make it perfect, delightful, and smooth.

Help me also to walk in the light of Your truth (Ephesians 1:18-23).

Now to Him who is able to do exceedingly abundantly above all that we ask or think, according to the power that works in us, to Him be glory in the

church by Christ Jesus to all generations, forever and ever Amen (Ephesians 3:20–21).

WEEK 20 - AGE OF YOUR LITTLE ONE

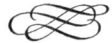

Week 20 - From the Date of Conception
Week 22 - From the Date of Your Last Period

At this stage, your little one has developed eyebrows, eyelids, and fingernails.

The baby also begins to develop brain cells at a fast rate, which continues for the next 12 weeks.

If your little one is a boy, his testes will have formed and begun their descent into the scrotum. If your little one is a girl, her mammary glands in the breasts begin to form.

Your little one continues practicing swallowing with the amniotic fluid and absorbing their nutrients as well as from the placenta.

His/her bones are becoming stronger. Though your little one's eyes are formed, they are without the pigment and remain shut until the 28th week.

. . .

Prayer

Gracious Lord, thank You for the beautiful miracle You are growing inside of me and that all Your works are good and perfect.

Thank You for perfecting the complex network of brain cells in my little one so that s/he functions perfectly. I pray that my little one will also connect with Your awesome grace and glory with ease.

May s/he know You even at a young age and be a man or woman after your heart.

All your children shall be taught by the Lord,

And great shall be the peace of your children (Isaiah 54:13).

WEEK 21 - AGE OF YOUR LITTLE ONE

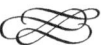

Week - 21 From the Date of Conception
Week - 23 From the Date of Your Last Period

At this stage, your little one can suck in preparation for breastfeeding. S/he also moves around inside the womb and uses his/her sense of hearing for orientation.

Your baby's eyeballs have now fully developed but remain closed for protection. The baby begins to produce insulin through his/her fully developed pancreas, which will later facilitate the breaking down of sugar.

Your baby's lungs are continuing to develop for post-birth, and s/he can clearly hear your voice and sounds from your surroundings. Continue to speak God's truths over your child. Your little one continues to flex his/her muscles whilst moving around and somersaulting.

Prayer
Father of glory, I thank You because You are

faithful to Your Word to perfect all that has been committed into Your hands.

I commit my little one into Your hands once again in full knowledge that Your mercies are new every morning. I pray that the environment of my womb will continue to be a source of sustenance, nourishment, and protection for my little one.

I thank You for the perfect functioning of the pancreas and that there will be no diabetes in either me or my little one. Thank You for my little one's strong and healthy lungs. Thank You that Your grace will abundantly carry us through to full term in good health. Thank You that I can be confident to receive all I ask in prayers.

"Ask, and it will be given to you; seek, and you will find; knock, and it will be opened to you" (Matt 7:7).

WEEK 22 - AGE OF YOUR LITTLE ONE

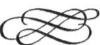

Week 22 - From the Date of Conception
Week 24 - From the Date of Your Last Period

At this stage, your little one is continuing to add flesh to bone and fill up the room in your womb.

The amniotic fluid, which helps the baby move around in the womb, cushions the baby and regulates his/her temperature. Permanent tooth buds are present in your little one's gums.

Your baby's lungs are also developing respiratory functions, and s/he continues to practise breathing in the amniotic fluid which helps prepare him/her to breathe in air. Your little one will also have developed sleeping patterns, so s/he will be active and then fall asleep.

Prayer

Heavenly Father, thank You for another week with this bundle of joy You have placed in my care. I am trusting You to infuse me with strength, resilience, and good health to bring this miracle to full term.

Thank You that You are providing my little one with healthy functioning lungs and other organs.

Thank You for the right level of amniotic fluid for his/her protection as well as my body functions.

Thank You that You will breathe the breath of life into my little one's lungs as s/he enters the world.

I thank You because You are prospering my health and soul and will keep prenatal and postnatal depression far from my soul.

Beloved, I pray that you may prosper in all things and be in health, just as your soul prospers
   (3 John 1:2).

WEEK 23 - AGE OF YOUR LITTLE ONE

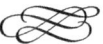

Week 23 - From the Date of Conception
Week 25 - From the Date of Your Last Period

If you're based in the UK and this is your first child, you are due for another appointment.

At this stage, your little one continues to add weight and strength. His/her little hands are fully formed.

Blood vessels are forming in the lungs, and the baby's nostrils begin to open to facilitate breathing. The baby's hearing is becoming sharper and can recognise the familiar voices of loved ones.

Your little one's nerve endings are continuing to develop, causing your little one to respond to stimuli. Your little one's eyes are developing underneath the lid, causing your little one to respond to light.

Prayer

Creator of heaven and earth, I bring You

praises today for the wonderful works of Your hands that are bringing me so much joy.

I thank You for the continuing work of your mighty hands in the formation of my little one. May my little one master Your voice as You graciously lead him/her along the paths of righteousness.

And may my little one respond to the light of your glory. May his/her lungs be always filled with praises to the glorious God we serve (John 10:27).

> **Though I walk in the midst of trouble, You will revive me;**
> **You will stretch out Your hand**
> **Against the wrath of my enemies,**
> **And Your right hand will save me.**
> **The Lord will perfect that which concerns me;**
> **Your mercy, O Lord, endures forever;**
> **Do not forsake the works of Your hands**
> **(Psalm 138:7–8).**

WEEK 24 - AGE OF YOUR LITTLE ONE

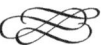

Week 24 - From the Date of Conception
Week 26 - From the Date of Your Last Period

Your little one's eyes may open this week. The baby's five senses are now alert.

The uterus is expanding, which allows light to filter in, so your little one is aware of darkness and light. Air sacs continue to develop in the lung area that will later expand with air.

Your little one now has regular sleeping and waking patterns. The baby's bone and spinal structure continues to strengthen.

Your little one may even start to suck his/her thumb for comfort and to strengthen his oral-motor skills.

Prayer

Heavenly Father, thank You for the beautiful eyes that You have given my little one; may my little one's eyes gravitate toward that which is good.

May my little one's vision be filled with the light of Your glory and view life from Your perspective. May he/she see life's challenges with boldness, courage, and with the knowledge of Your constant presence.

Thank You for blessing my baby with healthy lungs, strong bones, and a healthy sleeping pattern. By faith I receive Your perfect bloodline freely given in your new covenant for my little one (Matthew 7:7-8).

Likewise He also took the cup after supper, saying, "This cup is the new covenant in My blood, which is shed for you" (Luke 22:20).

WEEK 25 - AGE OF YOUR LITTLE ONE

Week 25 - From the Date of Conception
Week 27 - From the Date of Your Last Period

At this stage, your little one continues to grow in length and weight. Your baby continues practicing how to breathe by breathing in amniotic fluid.

His/her hearing is also continuously improving as s/he recognises familiar voices and sounds. Your baby's skin looks wrinkled from being in the amniotic fluid but will smooth out within a few weeks after birth.

Your little one can enter REM sleep and may even dream.

Prayer

Precious Lord of glory, thank You for another week where You have kept both me and my little one safe, nourished, and in good health.

Thank You for breathing the breath of life into my little one and for perfecting his/her breathing. I pray that my little one will not suffer from any form of breathing disorder.

Thank You that You give my little one sound sleep both now and after delivery. Thank You for filling my little one's mind with heavenly dreams and your angelic presence pre- and post-delivery.

I pray that Your abiding presence would be near us in the hour of delivery. Thank You for keeping us both healthy and removing all forms of complications pre- and post-birth. Thank You for strengthening my body to bring my little one to full term (Isaiah 41:10).

When you lie down, you will not be afraid;
   Yes, you will lie down and your sleep will be sweet (Proverbs 3:24).

CHAPTER 3

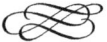

Third Trimester - Chapter 3

A Mother's Prayers

PART IV

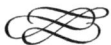

A Mother's Prayers

WEEK 26 - AGE OF YOUR LITTLE ONE

Week 26 - From the Date of Conception
Week 28 - From the Date of Your Last Period

If you're based in the UK, you are due another antenatal appointment.

At this stage, your baby's skin will begin to fill out where it was previously flat. Hair will be present on his/her head along with eyebrows and eyelashes.

Your little one's brain will develop the normal grooves on the surface area, and there will be an increase in brain tissue as other organs continue to mature. Your baby's eyes can blink and produce tears.

Your little one's heart has slowed down to around 140 beats per minute and strong enough to now be heard through a doctor's stethoscope.

*P*rayer
Dear Heavenly Father, thank You for Your

ongoing work in the development of this bundle of joy that You've placed lovingly in my care.

Thank You for giving my little one a wonderful healthy brain and the grace to have a beautiful and healthy life. Thank You for eyes that see Your truth and the purpose You've given my child to fulfil.

Thank You that my little one is gaining weight; may my little one always see him/herself as beautiful and perfectly created by Your loving hands.

May this child not be skewed in his/her thinking by unhealthy views. I pray that my little one will have unshakable confidence in what You think about him/her if ever this is in question.

May my little one's heart beat according to Your natural design all the days of his/her life.

I pray that my little one will develop a healthy strong heart that can stand the pressures of his/her generation and may my little one's heart always stay close to Yours.

"...but the people who know their God shall be strong, and carry out *great exploits*" (Daniel 11:32).

WEEK 27 - AGE OF YOUR LITTLE ONE

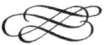

Week 27 - **From the Date of Conception**
Week 29 - From the Date of Your Last Period

Your little one is still growing in length and measures around 38.6 cm from crown to heel. His/her brain is gaining more grooves.

The baby's bones are beginning to gain strength, and you will need the intake of calcium to assist with the growth of his/her skeleton.

If you're unable to absorb dairy products you can find it in other foods rich in calcium, such as cannellini beans, broccoli, kale, and walnuts.

Your little one's senses will be developed enough to feel pain, be aware of movements in you, and control his/her body temperature.

As your little one's growth decreases the space in your womb, you may feel the force of the kicks enough to make you gasp and maybe even see the foot or hand shape pressed beneath your skin.

. . .

Prayer

Dear Heavenly Father, thank You again for this bundle of joy growing healthily and strong in my womb.

I pray that my little one will absorb enough calcium from me to develop strong and healthy bones for all the days of his/her life.

I pray that Your loving arms will keep sickness and bone diseases, including arthritis, far from my little one. I pray that like Moses and Caleb, who were strong in their old age, so shall my little one be (Joshua 14:12-15), (Deuteronomy 34:7).

Help me also to continue to eat and produce ample nutrients to nourish my little one. I also pray that my little one will always desire the sincere milk of Your Word to grow up in the knowledge of your love and salvation.

... as newborn babes, desire the pure milk of the word, that you may grow... (1Peter 2:2).

WEEK 28 - AGE OF YOUR LITTLE ONE

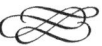

Week 28 - From the Date of Conception
Week 30 - From the Date of Your Last Period

At this stage, your baby is gaining weight and weighs on average around three pounds and can open and shut his/her eyes.

Growth in body length is much slower. Your little one's digestive tract and lungs are nearly fully developed, and his/her brain continues developing the grooves.

The layer of fat under your baby's skin will keep your baby warm after birth.

There will also be the presence of full hair on your little one's head. Though your little one is fully developed, the maturing of organs continues to take place.

Prayer

Dear loving Father, thank You for keeping my little one safe all this time in my womb.

Thank You for the provision of the nourishment in my

body that has enabled my little one to gain weight and be healthy.

Thank You, gracious Father, that You will breathe the breath of life into my little one at birth and that my little one's diaphragm and vital organs will work perfectly without complication.

Thank You, loving Father, as I trust You will be right here with us during delivery and all the days of our lives.

> **Let us therefore come boldly to the throne of grace, that we may obtain mercy and find grace to help in time of need (Hebrews 4:16).**

WEEK 29 - AGE OF YOUR LITTLE ONE

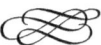

Week 29 - From the Date of Conception
Week 31 - From the Date of Your Last Period

If you're based in the UK and this is your first child, you are due for an antenatal appointment.

Your little one continues to increase his/her body fat and weight. At this stage, your little one's brain is rapidly developing nerve connections.

You will notice that your little one is sleeping for longer periods. Your little one's five senses are also developing further, and his/her eyes are recognising light and darkness as the iris continues to mature.

Your little one can now also recognise specific music and respond to it. S/he will now be urinating into the amniotic fluid and drinking the amniotic fluid. Your little one will also now be producing red blood cells from the bone marrow.

. . .

Prayer

Awesome God of glory, thank You for the presence of Your light and life in my womb.

Thank You that my little one is healthy, active, and strong because You are present with us.

I pray that my little one's personality will develop according to your awesome design and s/he will always be confident in who s/he is.

I pray that my little one will have an innate ability to connect with who s/he is despite any adverse thing life throws his/her way.

I pray that my little one will always have an unshakable confidence in who You are to him/her and therefore have confidence in who s/he is.

Train up a child in the way he should go,

And when he is old he will not depart from it (Proverbs 22:6).

WEEK 30 - AGE OF YOUR LITTLE ONE

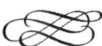

Week 30 - From the Date of Conception
Week 32 - From the Date of Your Last Period

Your baby is practising thumb sucking and swallowing, which prepares him/her for feeding.

Your little one is also still rapidly gaining weight for life outside the womb and, with less space to move around, s/he would have taken the head-down position for birth.

If your little one is bottom down or in breech position, do not worry as babies tend to change positions.

Your baby weighs approximately three and a quarter pounds.

Prayer

Heavenly Father, Creator of all things, thank You for the brilliance and intricacies You have put together in human life so that we can function and survive.

Thank You also that You are continuing to perfect the work You've started in my little one.

I pray that You will give my little one strength and a fighting spirit to overcome life's challenges with the excellence You've already imparted in the human body to fight diseases.

I pray that my little one will be resilient and have a persevering spirit, even from infancy. I join with all creation in giving glory and honour to Your holy name (Psalm 19:1-6).

I pray that my little one will master his/her sucking skills and the ability to feed healthily, and I pray for the grace to produce ample milk and wisdom to breastfeed correctly and commit to eating the right food to nourish my little one.

If breastfeeding is not my preferred method, I thank you Lord for providing other means of nourishing my child through modern science.

*L*ord, if this is my preferred method of feeding my child, but for any reason I am unable to produce milk, may you enfold me with your comforting arms and enable me to receive your grace to overcome this and seek other methods you've provided to nourish my little one.

I also pray that if my little one is in breech position that Your loving hands will also correct this to ease the birth.

There is therefore now no condemnation to those who are in Christ Jesus, who do not walk according to the flesh, but according to the Spirit (Romans 8:1).

WEEK 31 - AGE OF YOUR LITTLE ONE

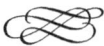

Week 31 - From the Date of Conception
Week 33 - From the Date of Your Last Period

Your little one has gained more weight and is now four pounds; s/he continues to fill the available space in your uterus and is now head down in the fetal position.

Moving around will be a bit restricted due to his/her size. Your little one's brain and nervous system have developed.

The antibodies you've passed down have enabled your little one to develop his/her own immune system.

His/her bones continue to grow stronger, and the skull is still soft with bony plates that overlap to facilitate birth. The skull does not fuse until your little one is well over a year old.

Prayer

Loving Father, thank You that my little one is rapidly gaining weight in preparation for birth. I pray that my little one's immune system will work perfectly to fight infections, germs, and bacteria.

I thank You for a strong and healthy immune system pre- and post-birth.

Thank You that You will be right with me and my little one during delivery to comfort and deliver us from evil (Matthew 6:13). I thank You that Your Word promises me that when I'm weak, in you I am strong.

And He said to me, "My grace is sufficient for you, for My strength is made perfect in weakness." Therefore most gladly I will rather boast in my infirmities, that the power of Christ may rest upon me (2 Corinthians 12:9).

WEEK 32 - AGE OF YOUR LITTLE ONE

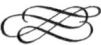

Week 32 - From the Date of Conception
Week 34 - From the Date of Your Last Period

If you're based in the UK, you are due for an antenatal appointment where information will be provided to you in preparation for labour.

At this stage, your baby weighs five pounds and is well acquainted with your voice, and his/her ears are sufficiently developed to recognise songs and nursery rhymes, now and post-birth.

If the baby is a boy, then his testicles will begin to appear in his scrotum. If this hasn't happened at birth, there is no need to worry, as this is not unusual and they will appear a little later.

Your little one's central nervous system and lungs are becoming fully developed.

. . .

Prayer

Heavenly Father, thank You for the life You've placed in my care and that s/he is developing further and getting ready to delight the world with his/her birth.

I commit my little one back into Your loving hands as You have the power of life to bring him/her forth as the perfect child You have created him/her to be.

I pray for healthy testicles, if my baby is a boy. I also pray for a healthy nervous system, and strong and perfect lungs for his/her first cry to be a cry that praises You for Your wonderful works that my soul knows so well.

I will praise You, for I am fearfully and wonderfully made;
    Marvellous are Your works,
    And that my soul knows very well (Psalm 139:14).

WEEK 33 - AGE OF YOUR LITTLE ONE

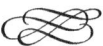

Week 33 - From the Date of Conception
Week 35 - From the Date of Your Last Period

Your little one is continuing to gain weight, weighs five and a half pounds, and his/her skin is filling out and looks smooth due to the fat building up to keep him/her warm after birth.

Your little one's activity will be reduced due to limited space in the womb and will move further down your pelvis.

Your little one's lungs are now fully developed, and his/her liver is fully functioning; growth is what's left.

Prayer

Loving Father, thank You for bringing us this far along the journey. I pray that my little one will gain the right amount of weight that will be in sync with passing through my birth canal.

I pray that if it is better for me to have a Caesarian section that you will give the doctors the wisdom and attention to details to know. I pray for grace to sleep at night, as delivery draws near, and grace to overcome fatigue.

I thank You that my little one's lungs are fully developed and ready to breathe in air after delivery.

I thank You for my little one's healthy liver that is fully capable of processing waste. Thank You that You have perfected all my little one's organs.

Thank You that I can place my trust in Your unfailing love to keep me strong and healthy to deliver and look after my little one. Thank You that, even as an infant, You have created strength within my little one to overcome challenges.

"Shall I bring to the time of birth, and not cause delivery?" says the Lord.

"Shall I who cause delivery shut up the womb?" says your God (Isaiah 66:9).

WEEK 34 - AGE OF YOUR LITTLE ONE

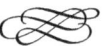

Week 34 - From the Date of Conception
Week 36 - From the Date of Your Last Period

If you're based in the UK, you're due an antenatal appointment where information will be provided to you about caring for your baby after birth.

At this stage, your little one weighs 6 pounds and will be 13½ inches in length. Your little one's systems are fully functioning except for the digestive system, which takes over a year to be fully developed.

Your little one is considered to have reached full term and is likely to move into the birth position head first, but you may not be in labour yet.

If your little one moves into position bottom first, then the baby will deliver breech. The midwife/practitioner has options and should assist with your decision of how you want to give birth.

Your begins to shed the lanugo hair that covers his/her body and the vernix substance into the amniotic fluid.

Your little one will swallow this and store it in his/her

bowels as meconium, which will form the baby's first stool post-birth.

Prayer

Heavenly Father, I thank You for protecting my little one and me up to this stage. I pray that as my little one prepares to be birthed that You will guide my little one to be correctly positioned.

I pray that there will not be a breech, and my little one will make safe entry into the world because You will be right there with us, championing my little one's birth.

Thank You for breathing into my little one's lungs Your breath of life. I pray against any complications with the umbilical cord, my little one, and my body. I pray that my little one will have a perfect bowel movement (Psalm 18:4-7, 27:1).

The Lord is my light and my salvation;
    Whom shall I fear?
    The Lord is the strength of my life;
    Of whom shall I be afraid? (Psalm 27:1).

WEEK 35 - AGE OF YOUR LITTLE ONE

Week 35 - From the Date of Conception
Week 37 - From the Date of Your Last Period

Your little one is continuing to grow, though at a slower rate and weighs around six and a half pounds.

If you're leaking amniotic fluid it is crucial that you inform your midwife or doctor.

Your little one will begin to flex his or her facial muscles by making various facial expressions and will also be able to identify and move toward light.

Your little one will have developed a pattern of movement that will continue until birth. Let your midwife or practitioner know if you notice any change.

***P*rayer**

Loving Father, I thank You for bringing us closer to my date of delivering this little bundle of joy You've placed in my care.

I thank You that my little one is healthy, strong, and

adding weight daily. I thank You that Your presence calms and comforts my little one so that s/he feels safe, loved, and valued.

Thank You for filling my little one with Your joy and may s/he be filled with a healthy zest for life.

Thank You for Your presence with us to prepare us and be with us in the hour of our delivery. Thank you for Your loving peace that rests upon me, keeping me from being anxious.

You are my hiding place;
 You shall preserve me from trouble;
 You shall surround me with songs of deliverance **(Psalm 32:7).**

WEEK 36 - AGE OF YOUR LITTLE ONE

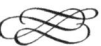

Week 36 - From the Date of Conception
Week 38 - From the Date of Your Last Period

At this stage if you are in the UK, you are due another antenatal appointment to discuss the possibility of your pregnancy continuing over 41 weeks and the options available to you.

Your little one is ready to be born with all his/her organs functioning well. Your little one will weigh an average of seven pounds.

Your little one continues to shed the vernix substance that has protected his/her skin in the amniotic fluid as well as the fine hair that has covered his/her skin.

Prayer

Mighty Father, thank You again for Your loving kindness and protection over our lives.

Thank You for shining Your light of glory on our lives as we prepare for delivery.

I thank You that my little one has learned to swallow, Thank You for the grace to love, and wisdom to care for my little one outside the womb. I pray that the delivery process will not be a lengthy ordeal.

I pray that the midwives, doctors and nurses who will be performing the delivery will be filled with Your grace, strength, excellence, discernment, and wisdom.

I also pray for good rest and strength for me as my body prepares for delivery. Please fill my heart with your peace and help me to trust you with every detail.

"Ask, and it will be given to you; seek, and you will find; knock, and it will be opened to you. For everyone who asks receives, and he who seeks finds, and to him who knocks it will be opened" (Matthew 7:7-8).

WEEK 37 - AGE OF YOUR LITTLE ONE

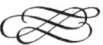

Week 37 - From the Date of Conception
Week 39 - From the Date of Your Last Period

Your little one will have limited space to move around in your womb at this stage. All your little one's organs are fully mature.

The lungs, which are the last to fully mature, are now producing surfactant, which helps the baby's airways to remain open to breathe after birth.

Your little one's skin is thickening. The infant will now weigh around seven and a half pounds. Your little one's brain is still rapidly growing.

The placenta will continue to supply oxygen and nutrients until your baby is born. Once your little one takes a first breath, his/her own heart will begin to function and transport oxygen and nutrients to him/her.

. . .

Prayer

Almighty Father in heaven, thank You for bringing my little one to full term.

I am trusting that You will also see us through a safe delivery.

I thank You for the umbilical cord that has been a source of sustenance for my little one; I pray that it will not be a source of danger during birth, and I pray that Your loving hands will move it to the right position.

I thank You for my little one's skin that is growing thicker layers; I pray that you will remove skin discomfort.

The Lord is my shepherd;
   I shall not want (Psalm 23:1).

WEEK 38 - AGE OF YOUR LITTLE ONE

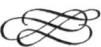

Week 38 - From the Date of Conception
Week 40 - From the Date of Your Last Period

If you are in the UK you are due another antenatal appointment, if this is your first baby.

Your little one now weighs around seven and a half pounds, and movement is restricted as s/he has filled out.

It is not unusual for your due date to have passed at this stage and your baby is just fine.

You are considered full term up to 42 weeks. Growth of your little one in the womb is all done at this stage.

It will take about three years for your little one's skull to completely fuse together. The skull overlaps to enable birth, so don't be surprised if your little one is born with his/her head looking cone-like as it will reshape itself after birth.

Your little one will be born with over 70 skills and reflexes to begin his/her life journey.

Your little one should now be positioned with head down, knees against nose in preparation for birth. Some pregnancies can go over 40 weeks, and in such cases, your midwife/practitioner will keep an eye on you and run tests to make sure your little one is okay.

Your midwife will also advise you of the options available to accelerate the birth. If your pregnancy is high-risk, then your labour will be induced.

When your little one is born, your midwife will clear his/her airways and examine their vital signs and check responsiveness. You will hear the long-awaited sound of your baby's first cry. Your little one will only be able to see 2.5 cm in front of him/her but will recognise your voice and your partner's.

Prayer

Heavenly Father, I lift my eyes to You as I approach the hour of delivery. I thank You for Your promise in Your infallible Word that You will neither slumber nor sleep during my delivery and that you will deliver my little one and me from all evil.

Please see us safely on the other side of the birthing process (Psalm 121).

Father, I thank You that You will be the first to welcome my little one into the world with Your breath of life, purpose, protection, and joy. I thank You that You have given my little one everything needed to survive in this world.

I pray that You will keep me healthy and nourished to take care of this bundle of joy You have placed in my care. Please give me the wisdom, understanding, and patience to know my little one's needs and nurture them.

I pray for emotional intelligence for me and my partner to discern challenges that need medical assistance.

Help my partner and me to enjoy every stage of my little one's development post-birth and choose to make good memories at each stage of his/her development outside the womb.

I pray that my little one develops a healthy sleep pattern, and may we have the resilience to forbear if this takes time. (If breastfeeding is my choice), I pray that my breasts will produce ample milk, nourishment, and antibodies for my little one.

And if I choose an alternative method, I pray that you will bless that means as well, for nothing is impossible with you. Help my partner and me to champion my little one to fulfil Your purpose for his/her life. Amen!

..."My soul magnifies the Lord,
And my spirit has rejoiced in God my Saviour..."
(Luke 1:46–47).

WEEK 39 - AGE OF YOUR LITTLE ONE

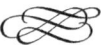

Week 39 - From the Date of Conception
Week 41 - From the Date of Your Last Period

At this stage, if you have not yet given birth, you will be due another antenatal appointment if you're based in the UK.

Your midwife or doctor will carry out a number of checks and discuss options with you for labour induction.

Your baby is doing well, but your midwife or doctor will ensure that the baby is safely delivered no later than two weeks past the due date.

It is not unusual for pregnancies to last over 41 weeks and the baby may well not be late, but the due date might not have been right to start with. Your little one is finding less space to move around, but you will still feel movements and kicks.

Your little one will produce hormones to induce labour when s/he is ready for birth.

. . .

Prayer

Heavenly Father, I thank you that you are with me and my little one and have protected us both up till now.

I thank you that you will provide comfort and grace for me, as I might find this last week going slowly, and sometimes sleeping may be a bit challenging.

I pray for the comfort of the Holy Spirit to enfold me at this time so that I can maintain a peaceful demeanour as I await the delightful entrance of my little one into the world and our family.

Fill me with deep and unconditional love for my little one, just as you have, and always will, love me.

From the end of the earth I will cry to You,

When my heart is overwhelmed;

Lead me to the rock that is higher than I (Psalm 61:2).

WEEK 40 - AGE OF YOUR LITTLE ONE

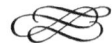

Week 42

For the mothers that have reached 42 weeks, it's perfectly okay and normal. Your little one's arrival is imminent.

Prayers

Dear loving and heavenly Father, I thank you for your promise to be with me always and that you're faithful and true to your words. I pray that you would give me wisdom to make the right decision with respect to the induction of my little one, if it is necessary.

I pray for your strength as I wait on you Lord.

Help me not to be weary at this stage when my little one is due anytime from now.

May the blessed assurance of your presence calm all my fears and prepare me physically, mentally and psychologically for the birthing process.

I thank you that your perfect love is casting out all fear as

I wear the helmet of salvation and choose to think on faith-filled thoughts.

*B*less my little one with strength, perseverance, and resilience as s/he makes their journey through the birth canal to life outside the womb. I pray for divine health, peace, and protection.

"Before she was in labor, she gave birth;
   Before her pain came,
   She delivered a male child (Isaiah 66:7).

GOOD READING?

Thank you for letting me be part of your journey through A Mother's Prayers.

If this devotional was helpful to you, **please leave a review**, as it will help make this book visible to someone else who might need it.

Additionally, if you would like to be informed of other book launches and promotions by me, you can sign up to my Reader's List with the link below, where you will receive my free poem called *"The Voice Within".*

www.joanneswellofpearls.com/sign-up

I will never spam you and you can unsubscribe at anytime.

FURTHER READING

Further Reading

Francis and Judith MacNutt, *Praying for your Unborn Child*, Hodder & Stoughton, 2011

Ina May Gaskin, *Ina May's Guide to Childbirth*, Bantam Doubleday Dell, 2003

BIBLIOGRAPHY

Curtis, Glade B., MD, MPH and Judith Schuler, MS. *Your Pregnancy: Week by Week*. 8th ed. Your Pregnancy Series. Boston: DaCapo Lifelong Books, 2016.

"Kid's Health: The Web's Most Visited Site About Children's Health." KidsHealth.com. 1995-2018. www.kidshealth.org.

"Pregnancy Week by Week." Baby Center LLC. 1997-2018. https://www.babycenter.com/pregnancy-week-by-week.

"Pregnancy Week by Week." Bounty.com. 2001-2017. http://www.bounty.com/pregnancy-and-birth/pregnancy/pregnancy-week-by-week.

"What to Expect: The #1 Pregnancy & Parenting Brand." whattoexpect.com. https://www.whattoexpect.com.

"Your Pregnancy and Baby Guide" www.nhs.uk
   https://www.nhs.uk/conditions/pregnancy-and-baby/

antenatal-appointment-schedule/#eight-to-14-weeks-dating-scan

ACKNOWLEDGMENTS

I would like to first thank Father God, for giving me the insight, courage and gentle nudges to persist and bring this dream to reality.

He also blessed me so much by bringing very useful networks and resources along my way that has played a huge part in successfully completing and self-publishing this book.

I would like to thank my editor, Julie Cantrell for her assistance and very useful comments in the editing process, to which I am extremely grateful.

I would also like to thank my editor Helen Jones for her meticulous attention to details in the proofreading stage, her insightful comments and assistance with the layout of the manuscript. Very grateful to have found her online.

I'd would like to thank my friend Donna Kajita, for her

assistance in proof-reading and helpful comments, which I consider to be a blessing - You truly rose to the challenge!

Lastly, I'd like to thank my friends who helped me read over the manuscript.